Pilates for Beginners

RicTamily Royalties

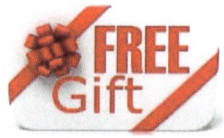

Want Priority Access to FREE eBooks?

As we release NEW eBooks, we offer them for FREE for a limited time. You will be the FIRST one to know when they are FREE. Join 1000's of insiders who are getting access to FREE Kindle book promotions weekly.

Click HERE for FREE additional material and FREE eBooks- www.rictamilypublishing.com

---

You Will Also Get Free Access to Additional Materials for this Book

Click HERE for FREE additional material and FREE eBooks- www.rictamilypublishing.com

Dedication

To our three blessings that have made RicTamily complete and continue to grow together in His loving embrace.

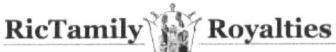

Contents

Chapter I: Getting to know Pilates

There are many forms of exercise that are popular nowadays. These include yoga, Tai' Chi, Chi-gong and Pilates. In this book, we will discover more about Pilates, its benefits and the forms of exercise that can be used in maintaining a healthy body with lean and developed muscles.

Pilates and its History

This is a method of conditioning the body invented by Joseph Pilates. It is a technique of having the body and mind fuse, leading to improvement in posture, strength, flexibility and an overall change in how a person feels about his or her body.

This program was originally designed as a rehabilitation program for the veterans of World War I as contrology or mat work. The developer designed it after his apprenticeship and study of Ancient Roman and Greek physical regimens, Zen and Yoga. Precise movements were formed because of his belief in the connection between mind and body. The movements are focused on the form and control of the entire body. Through its principles, a person experiences the transformation of the body as a whole.

The difference between other exercises and Pilates is that it develops multiple groups of muscles simultaneously. Joseph Pilates believed that building a strong core or powerhouse was essential. This core is comprised of the muscles under the shoulder blades, those surrounding the rib cage and down to the gluteals and hips.

The Core

The integration of the trunk, pelvis and shoulder girdle is the way to achieve core control. The techniques involved in Pilates paves the way to developing physical energy from the core to manifest the movements of the limbs. All movements are focused on muscle control. Each movement was created for a certain purpose; therefore, each is a contributor to the success as a whole.

The exercises not only develop weak muscles, but enhance the elasticity of the muscles as well as the balance of the body.

Materials

Most of the movements under the Pilates are mat exercises, meaning they are performed on the ground. However, there are numerous Pilate's machines that can aid in exercising. The difference is, in mat works, your own body weights acts as the resistance. On the other hand, machines facilitate increased intensity because of the additional resistance from the spring.

Chapter II: Pilates Principles

In order to keep track of obtaining certain objectives, principles must be followed. The principles were designed to be followed and to guide the performance of each exercise.

The Six Principles of Pilates

There are over 500 exercises related to Pilates and each exercise was rooted from the following principles.

Centering

The center of the core is the most important part of the body. It is also the area of focus in Pilate's exercises. It was believed that the energy needed to do the exercises correctly comes from the core center. The energy flows outside the body and manifests in the movements of the limbs. Through the core center, a strong foundation and stability can be maintained.

Breathing

One of the most important principles knows how to breathe with precision, concentration and control. The developer believed that in order to awaken the cells in our body, blood circulation is necessary. In order to have a good blood circulation, oxygen must be distributed throughout the body and wastes shall be eliminated.

The developer also believed that the proper oxygenation of the muscles shall be achieved through thorough and full inhalation and exhalation. Inhalation requires the maintenance of engagement while exhalation requires the engagement of pelvic muscles, together with the abdomen and the rib cage.

Precision

The focus of the movements in Pilates requires precision. The intrinsic value of each movement and their purpose are forsaken if there is no precision. This shall be the second nature of each practitioner of Pilates.

Concentration

Quality is more important than quantity. When doing a precise movement, one must have an effective concentration. By concentrating, you will become aware of how your body feels. It is also important that your mind and body act as one to produce precise movements.

Control

The purpose of every movement is to enhance muscle control. Thus, doing sloppy and uncontrolled movements are not effective in achieving such purpose. Work becomes more efficient when there is control and balance in the body.

Flow

Efficiency shall be continuous. The transitions between exercises must be smooth. This will improve stamina and strength. This will also allow the body to master safe and efficient movements.

Chapter III: Why do men and women practice Pilates?

To get involved in an exercise program means that you have a goal. These goals will help endure the pain. Each person definitely has driving force that will help them achieve their wants or needs.

Why do men practice Pilates?

There are many reasons for doing Pilates; however, these are the most common ones.

Building strength and power

The Pilates focus is promoting core strength and letting it flow outward to the limbs. By using core strength, performance is maximized and power is built. The practitioner of Pilates found it easy to perform explosive movements more efficiently. The strong foundation of strength and power is core stability.

Developing neglected muscles

We cannot deny the fact that most of the muscles in the body are undeveloped. The muscles that we need in our daily activities, such as those in the arms and legs, are stronger than other muscles. In doing Pilates, the movements help to divert effort from primary muscles and tone the neglected ones. The agonist muscles, supporting muscles, become more developed while doing Pilates.

Enhancing Flexibility

Flexibility is often based on muscle mass. More muscle masses tend to decrease flexibility. However, by practicing Pilates, flexibility is enhanced. This will lead to a lower chance of acquiring muscles strains and injuries.

Improved Stamina

Men who work jobs that require great stamina can benefit from Pilates. Studies have shown that middle aged men who practice Pilates have significantly increased upper-body and abdominal strength and endurance.

Why do women practice Pilates?

While men do Pilates for physical advancement, most women do this for health, style and beauty. The following are the most common reasons women do Pilates.

Help in the preparation for pregnancy

For a pregnant woman, Pilates will be of great help in strengthening the pelvic floor, back and tummy muscles without giving stress to other joints. There are several Pilates classes conducted especially for pregnant women. The benefit is increased function in the muscles that may give rise to problems during pregnancy.

Pilates also promotes balance. This will help you walk and stand properly without tripping or falling due to your baby bump. It also helps in learning proper breathing that is necessary in labor.

Full body sculpting

The most common workout for women focuses on sole cardiovascular exercises. However, this type of workout does not eliminate excessive calories in the body. The true exercise must be a combination of strength enhancement and cardiovascular endurance.

Pilates can give you a full body workout, which is a must in sculpting your body. You might feel that your whole body is at sore when you first take classes, but this will eventually shape up your body.

Chapter IV: Workouts for Beginners

In every engagement, you must start with the basics. This will help your body to adopt in the movements. This will help lessen the risk of injury or strain.

The warm up

Starting Position - Constructive Rest - Neutral Spine

This will be the first position to perform prior to other fundamental exercises.

You must lie on your back, arms by your side. Bend your knees with feet flat on the floor about a hip distance apart. Inhale and exhale. Use your ABS to press your spine onto the floor.

Head nod

This is an extension to obtain a lengthened spine. This is an essential part of numerous Pilate's exercises involving articulation of the spine.

In performing this, start with the neutral spine position. To lengthen your spine, inhale. Then, tilt your chin towards your chest without removing your head from the mat.

Exhale to return to the first position. Repeat the cycle again.

Arms over

This focuses on the alignment of the body. This also challenges the torso by lifting the arms overhead. This also enables the enhancement of the shoulder joint range.

To perform this motion, start with the first position. Inhale as you bring your hands up to the ceiling. Exhale as you rest your arms on the floor behind you.

Repeat the cycle.
Basic movements for beginners

Pilates Hundreds

To start, lie on your back and bend your knees with your feet flat on the floor. Your arms should be at your side, palms down. Tilt your hips to contract your ABS, pushing down your lower back against the mat. Simultaneously, lift your head, neck, and shoulder blades off the floor. Continue while inhaling and exhaling slowly.

Lastly, pump your arms in an up and down motion by your sides, palms facing the floor. This should be done in a pressing motion.

Pilates Kneeling Rear Leg Raises

Start on knees and elbows on the mat, evenly distributing your weight. Your knees should be properly placed directly under your hip joints. Also, your elbows shall be directly under your shoulder sockets. Pull your belly button toward your spine.

Extend one leg. Your toes shall not touch the ground. Lift your leg as high as you can, this will make your back arch.

Switch legs and repeat.

Chapter V: Moves for Burning Calories

These are the movements used by women who want to achieve their desired body. These steps enable them to burn excessive calories in the body.

Swimming

The first step is to lie on your stomach with pubis firmly anchored in the mat, forehead down and inner thighs tightly pressed together. Your arms should be stretched forward as far as possible with the palms down and toes pointed. In a count of one, lift altogether your arms, chest, head and legs and hold.

Inhale and exhale normally while alternately lifting your arms and legs without touching the ground. Occasionally lift higher and reach longer for progress.

Crisscross

To start, lie on your back with your hands behind your lifted head, palm over another. Your knees should be bent tightly into your chest. As you inhale slowly, twist your torso to the left until your right elbow touches your left knee. Straighten your right leg and hold it a few inches above the mat. Exhale and do the same procedure on the other side.

Six sets of twists are recommended.

Jogging knees with heel ups

Your elbows shall be pinned to your sides and your ABS shall be pulled in and up as you begin lifting your knees in a hip height. After approximately 8 knee lifts, begin kicking your bottom using your heels. After that kicks, you have the option to continue another set or move on to the next exercise.

Leg Pull

To begin, sit tall and extend your legs straight, squeezing them tightly together. Your feet should be pointed. Rest your palms on the edge of the mat behind you with your fingers pointing inward. Put the pressure on your hands as you elevate your hips. Make your body look like a diagonal line from head to heels.

Inhale as you lift your right leg as high as possible without losing your balance. Exhale as you control your feet as they return to the mat.

Switch legs and repeat the steps.

Chapter VI: Pilates Moves for a Flat Stomach

Every woman wants good posture and a flat stomach. Here are some moves that will result in a flat stomach.

Saw

To perform this exercise, sit tall with your back straight and waist lengthened. Your arms should be opened straight out to your sides at shoulder level and form a "crack- a -walnut" figure between your shoulder blades. Your legs are open wider than your shoulders, together with a flexed foot from the ankles and an anchored bottom on the mat.

Inhale while you rotate your trunk to your left and round over your left knee, as you press your right hand against the out edge of your left foot. Lift your back arm as high as possible. Exhale as you slide your right hand to the outside of the left foot in sawing motions as you draw back in, creating diagonal opposition for your ABS.

Inhale as you return to the first position and perform three sets.

Double- leg stretch

Hug you're both knees into your chest with your head forward, lifted and your elbows wide.

Control your inhalation as you reach your legs forward and arms in backward position, each stretching in opposition, which draws your abdomen in deeply to support your spine. Slowly exhale as you return to the first position, with the knees hugged to chest. Expand your diaphragm to allow air to enter your lungs.

Repeat this six times.

Corkscrew

Lie on your back with your arms by your sides. Squeeze your legs tightly together.

As lift your legs overhead, inhale slowly. This will make you roll back until you balance yourself in the middle of your shoulder blades and the back of your arms.

Point your toes while you control your exhalation as you roll back to your spine, your body slightly leaning to the right. Circle your legs to the left as you inhale slowly, as you roll up to your left side. Scoop your ABS and lift your bottom. Shift directions and complete three sets.

Chapter VII: Pilates for Larger People

Women are conscious about their bodies; however, many women who are heavy are comfortable with their weight. Other plus-size women and men are working to lose weight and need a place to start. The following exercises are appropriate for the heavier population.

The Dart

Lie face down on the mat with legs and feet together. Place your arms at your sides and relax your shoulders.

Inhale deeply through your nostrils, and breathe towards the back of your nostrils. Remember to exhale through your mouth. This exercise requires 4 breaths.

Inhale as you open your chest and squeeze shoulders back. Exhale as you reach your hands towards your feet, simultaneously ending your upper body above the floor.

Inhale as you hold the position and lengthen your head and feet in opposite ways. Exhale as you return to your original position.

Pull Down

Grab your exercise band and hold it in place where you feel sufficient tension. Reach your arms over your head with your elbows slightly bent. After this, recheck the tension.

Inhale deeply through your nostrils, and breathe towards the back of your nostrils. Remember to exhale through your mouth. This exercise requires 4 breaths.

In preparing, you must inhale. Exhale as you pull down in front your head as you extend your upper body above the mat. Inhale as you hold this position as you lengthen your head and feet in opposite directions. Exhale as you return.

In performing this, you must keep an eye on your neck and shoulder alignment.

Chapter VIII: Pilates for a 6- pack

Male physique can potentially include a six- pack ABS. There are Pilates moves recommended to obtain and maintain six- pack.

Pelvic Bridge or Pelvic Curl

This exercise is often used a warm- up for abdominal muscles and the spine. It also develops the coordination of breathing and movement and promotes the lower body muscles.

Duration is 5 minutes.

To start, find neutral spine position.

You must breathe in into your chest, to your belly, and to your pelvic floor. You must breathe out of your pelvic area, belly and chest.

Exhale as you tilt your pelvic involving the abdominal muscles and pull your belly button down towards your spine. Continue this action to press the lower spine using your ABS.

Inhale as you press your feet down, enabling your tail bone to begin to curl towards the ceiling. Raise your hips, then your lower spine and finally, the middle spine. Keep your legs parallel all the time.

Repeat this three to five times.

The Roll Up Ab Pilates Exercise

Start by lying on your back with extended arms along the floor above your head.

Inhale while squeezing your buttock and inner thighs together. Flex your feet. After this, exhale as you roll up, gesturing your straightened arms beyond you. Stretch your arms forward as you place your fingertips, beyond your toes.

Repeat exercise 10-15 times.

Chapter IX: Strengthening the legs and back with Pilates

As we age, our back and leg muscles are the most affected. In order to strengthen them, these are the recommended Pilate exercises.

Back Bow Crossover

To start, lie face down on the mat with your arms and legs extended in a straight line. Place an object like dumbbell on the floor above your head at your arm's length. Place both of hands on the left of the object, allowing your body to arch to the left.

Contract your core muscles as you lift your arms and legs up and above to exaggerate the arch to the right. Lower your hands slowly to the right side of the object and let your hands and feet momentarily touch the ground before making another arch to the opposite side.

Do this repetitively for a period of time.

Pilates Back Bows

Lie face down on the mat and extend your arms above your head.

Inhale while contracting your legs and core. Exhale while lifting your chest and arms up above as high as you can.

Inhale as you lower your body to the ground slowly as your arms and chest briefly touch the ground before repeating the steps. Continue without permitting your core to relax.

Lunges

Stand with one foot in front of the other, wide stance as if each foot is placed on a railroad track. Lower toward the ground by bending the knees and lift back up. Repeat several times on each leg. Whatever your weight may be, it is significant for a single leg. This thigh and butt exercise is a great way to tone the muscles in the legs and build lean muscles.

Chapter X: Pilates: The Claims

The following are the claims relating to Pilates exercises.

Leaner and longer muscles

The flexibility of the muscles is increased, which gives rise to the feeling of a longer muscle. Leaner muscles are part of the output of any activity.

Improved postural issues

Postural improvements do not pertain to height, but rather to the strength of the core and the purposeful lifting of each individual. Posture will improve with strength and consciousness to sitting and standing tall on a consistent basis.

Increased stability, peripheral mobility and core strength

Core strength is tested using a device called EMG or Electromyography. One of the studies tested the effects of Pilates in the three superficial core muscles, namely rectus abdominis or the ABS, external oblique's or the sides of the abdomen and rectus femoris or the muscles in legs which are used during sit-ups. Findings confirmed that these muscles were positively enhanced by Pilate's exercises. They gained a higher EMG value compared to the general requirements.

Due to the promotion of flexibility, Pilates exercises results to peripheral mobility or mobility the limbs.

Injury prevention

Building core strength can reduce the likeliness of falls and promotes a faster recovery if a fall is encountered.

Enhancing functional fitness and ease of movements

Functional fitness is defined as how the power, endurance, strength and flexibility that influences your daily living functions. As Pilates makes your muscles stronger, daily functions are improved. Physical chores may be completed with more ease and the likelihood of injury is reduced.

Some other claims

These include: balancing strength and flexibility, heightens body awareness, easy on joints with little or no impact. Pilates can be modified to fit everyone, including rehab patients and elite athletes. Pilates compliments other methods of exercise, improves sports performance, and lastly, improves circulation, coordination and balance.

Checkout Other Books by RicTamily Royalties

Anti-Cancer Diet: The Ultimate Guide in Fighting Cancer, Lowering Cancer Risk and Achieving Optimum Health

Gout Cure: Your Ultimate and Comprehensive Guide in Treating Gout Permanently

Anger, Stress and Fear: Your Personal Guide in Controlling Anger, Managing Stress and Overcoming Fear

Pilates for Beginners: The Essential Guide to Total Body Fitness, Strong Muscles and Lean Body

Stop Self-Sabotaging and Shift your Paradigm to Success: Your Ultimate Guide in Start Living the Life You Always Wanted

Chakras for Beginners: The Ultimate Guide to Balancing Chakras, Radiating Positive Energies and Strengthening Auras

The Ultimate Guide to Financial Freedom: Achieve Wealth, Attain Success and Manage Your Debt like the Rich

The True Nature of Intelligence: Musing on the Sumerian Culture from a Christian Perspective

The Ad: A Mail-Order Bride Romance Series

Gilgamesh - King in Quest for Immortality: An Extra-Biblical Proof for the Genesis Flood

Liver Cleanse and Detox Diet: The Ultimate Guide in Cleansing the Body, Eliminating Toxins and Losing Weight!

Top Ten Pets for Children: Tips on Care and Proper Choice for Your Child

Teeth Healing Through Oil Pulling: The Complete Guide in Natural Oral Care through the Benefits of Oil Pulling

Herbal Soap Making: How to Make Homemade Soaps that clean and Nurture the Body

10 Things You Need to Know About Ebola: Facts about the Virus, Symptoms, Quarantine and Prevention

Please Leave a Review

If you enjoyed this book, we would really appreciate it if you could leave us a positive REVIEW

P.S. You can CLICK HERE to go directly to the book page and leave your review and/or purchase our other books above. Alternately, you can copy and paste this address into your browser ---
http://amzn.to/1wCj3OE

THE END

www.ingramcontent.com/pod-product-compliance
Lightning Source LLC
Chambersburg PA
CBHW050932290526
45792CB00002B/983